GLUTATHIONE

Your Body's Secret Healing Agent

Holly Fourchalk, PhD., DNM®, RHT, HT

CHOICES UNLIMITED

FOR

HEALTH & WELLNESS

DISCLAIMER

Every effort has been made by the author to ensure that the information in this book is as accurate as possible. However, it is by no means a complete or exhaustive examination of all information.

The author knows what worked for her and what has worked for others but no two people are the same and so the author cannot and does not render judgment or advice regarding a particular individual.

Further, because our bodies are unique any two individuals may experience different results from the same therapy.

The author believes in both prevention and the superiority of a natural non-invasive approach over drugs and surgery.

The information collected within comes from a variety of researchers and sources from around the world. This information has been accumulated in the Western healing arts over the past thirty years.

Research has shown that one of the top three leading causes of death in North America occurs because of the physician/pharmaceutical component of the scenario.

Perhaps the real leading cause of death and disability is a result of the lack of awareness of natural therapies. These therapies are well known to prevent and treat many common degenerative, inflammatory and oxidative diseases.

The author loves to research and loves to teach. This book is another attempt to increase awareness about health and the many options we have to bring the body back into a healthy balance.

Ever-increasing numbers of people are aware of healing foods and herbs, supplements and modalities but there are still far too many who are not. The fact that our physicians are part of this latter group makes healing even more challenging yet we are now seeing more and more laboratories around the world and more universities in and outside of the U.S. studying herbs, nutrition and various healing modalities with phenomenal success.

The unfortunate fact is, those who can profit from sickness and disease promote ignorance and the results are devastating.

It is not the intent of the author that anyone should choose to read this book and make decisions regarding their health or medical care based on ideas contained in this book.

It is the responsibility of the individual to find a health care practitioner to work with to achieve optimal health.

The author and publisher are not responsible for any adverse effects or consequences resulting from the use of any of the suggestions or information contained in the book but offer this material as information that the public has a right to hear and utilize at its own discretion.

To my Parents

For all their support and encouragement
My Dad for his ever-listening ear
My mother for her open mind

INDEX

INTRODUCTION

Fun Introduction to the Human Body

Our bodies are a wonderfully inter-dynamic, interdependent, complex system. Western medicine failed us miserably by attempting to get too reductionist about our bodies, as if one system, one organ, etc. can function in and of itself. Western medicine still does a moderately good job in the emergency room, although current statistics reveal that more than 70% of diagnoses made in the emergency room are incorrect.

Despite that, I was sure appreciative of the team that reconstructed my ankle (foot and leg) when I had an accident and smashed it.

I am also sure that the thousands of peoples whose lives are saved thanks to emergency rooms are also appreciative.

But the ultimate thanks for good health and healing goes to our bodies and their ability to function. Let's start with a little trivia on how inter-dependent the body is:

- No system can operate independent of all other systems.

1

- No tissue can operate independent of all other tissues and systems of the body.
- No organ can operate independent of all the systems, tissues and organs of the body.
- Even our cells are wonderfully complex, dependent on all the different components within the cells, bathed in the fluids that connect each cell with all the different aspects of the system.
- Even the inside and the outside of the body are intricately connected. Our gastro-intestinal tract is a complex tube that runs from the mouth to the anus. While this system lies within the body, when we go into the system, we are actually outside of the body. Yet our bodies are tremendously dependent on this system.
- Many will also argue that the brain and the mind are not synonymous but rather the mind is held within the energetic field around and within the body and that the brain is a reflection of what goes on in the mind. Yet, we all know that what goes on in the body can have a huge impact on the brain and the brain can have a massive impact on the mind.
- We all know that ultimately everything is made up of energy. People whose bodies have healed due to energetic medicine and those who work with energetic medicine are

particularly aware of how the mind and body can impact the energy fields and how the energy fields can impact the body.

These phenomenally intricate systems are not only connected with each other within the system but as mentioned above, with systems outside of the body, i.e., the gastro-intestinal system.

If we were really thorough, we would also be exploring how every system, organ, tissue, cell, organelle, molecule, atom, neutron, photon is ultimately just energy. We also have to explore all the different kinds of energies: potential energy, magnetic energy, electro-magnetic, quantum, kinetic, gravitational, thermal, chemical and elastic energy.

Alas, that is way too much for this little book. Before we move on to exploring glutathione, let's have some fun and take a quick glimpse at what all these components of the body need to organize and create constantly, without any knowledge, understanding or direction from us.

- We make 250 million red blood cells per second which last between 90-120 days.
- We have about 2.5 trillion of these cells at any given time.
- It takes one red blood cell about 20 seconds to circulate the body.
- You have about 5.6 liters or 6 quarts of blood

- platelets are one of the major components of blood – you make about 200 billion per day

50 different types of immune cells
- 90% of our immune system is in our gut

Over 100 known neurotransmitters
- a nerve impulse can travel at over 400 Km/hr or 25 m/hr
- brain has over 100 billion nerve cells
- the spinal cord has about 13,500 neurons
- the skin contains about 45 miles of nerves
- the skin contains about 1300 nerve cells

Over 50 known hormones
- hormones are the inter communicators between different systems in the body

Over 2,700 known enzymes in the human body
- enzymes regulate 10s of thousands of biochemical functions
- enzymes combine co-enzymes to form nearly 100,000 various chemicals in the body
- 3 categories of enzymes: those found in food; those used to digest food; and those for all the other metabolic processes in the body

Seven categories of food enzymes
- Those that break down fats: lipases
- Those that break down proteins: proteases
- Those that break down fiber: cellulases
- Those that break down starch: amylases

- Those that break down grains: maltases
- Those that break down sugars: sucrases
- Your body requires over 20 different types of amino acids to make enzymes
- Any given cell has between 200-3000 enzymes

29 known types of collagen

- Found in: bones, cartilage, tendons, ligaments, skin, blood vessels, gut, hair, nails
- 206 bones: 29 bones in the skull
- Over 600 muscles
- About 100,000 hairs on the scalp

Constantly replicating 10^{12} cells in our bodies.
About 25 million new cells produced every second.

- Each cell contains: nucleus, nucleolus, ribosomes, vesicles, rough and smooth endoplasmic reticulum, Golgi apparatus, mitochondria, cytosol (the fluid), lysosomes, cytoskeleton, centrosome, cell membrane
- You shed about 600,000 particles of skin every hour
- You will lost about 105 pounds of skin by the age of 70
- You grow a new layer of skin every month
- One square inch of skin has about 3 million cells
- Overall the human skin has about 280,000 heat receptors
- Make about one liter of saliva per day

- A taste bud lasts about 10 days
- The cells of a taste bud lasts about 10 hours
- The tongue has about 10,000 taste buds
- Before their first birthday, babies will have dribbled about 255 pints of saliva
- Make between 100- 625 sweat glands per inch of human skin
- Your stomach produces a new layer of mucous lining every two weeks

And just as a side note, you burn more calories sleeping than you do watching TV. Why? Because typically during your sleep you are doing most of the repair work.

Our bodies have a working knowledge, capacity and ability to organize and direct that work that goes way beyond our comprehension. We are only just starting to understand it.

This is one of the many reasons Western medicine is so flawed. The way the Western medicine is presented actually makes us think that prescribed treatments can do a better job than our body already do but all prescriptions usually do is manage and mask symptoms using artificial synthetic toxic drugs. Further, these drugs end up depleting the very nutrients the body requires to function effectively.

When we consider that this is just the tip of the iceberg, we can begin to appreciate why our bodies require good healthy nutrients to keep our health at an optimal level.

When we become deficient in a given nutrient, the body has to start compensating. In fact, the body can compensate in thousands of different ways, protecting you from symptoms. Unfortunately, in Western culture, this has become a detriment. We keep feeding the body artificial foods, nutrient deficient foods, pasteurized, microwaved, processed foods – never mind all the toxins – and expect it to keep serving us well.

Then we go to a physician who prescribes toxic drugs that further deplete the body of its nutrients and mask the symptoms, which allows the underlying issues to continue to erode our health.

This type of ignorant, irresponsible functioning has led to our current state of overweight, hypertensive, arthritic, diabetic, fatigued, depressed state of "health". Or, more accurately, state of imbalance, disease and dysfunction.

But, it is possible to recover.

You wouldn't believe how many roles glutathione plays in this process...so let's now focus on glutathione.

ONE

What is Glutathione?

Glutathione is a fascinating molecule that your body creates in every cell. It certainly must be of interest to the scientific community considering that there are now over 100,000 Pubmed.com articles on glutathione. To give a context for this, there are just over 50,000 articles on Vitamin D and over 42,000 articles on Vitamin C.

Without sufficient glutathione, any given cell will die. We cannot absorb glutathione through food or supplementation as it breaks down in the stomach's hydrochloric acid and we lose some of the unstable components.

Even if it didn't break down, it is too large a molecule to pass through the cellular (phospholipid) membrane and there are no transport mechanisms to pass it through. So we are dependent on the cells to make it.

So, what is it? In biochemical terms, it is a tripeptide. This means that it has three amino acids: cysteine, glycine, and glutamate.

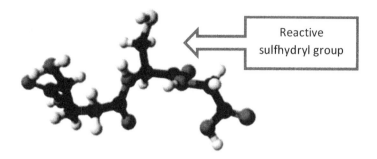

Reactive sulfhydryl group

Glutamic acid – cysteine – glycine

The cysteine amino acid also has a sulfhydryl or thiol group which allows it to act as an anti-oxidant. In addition, that cysteine is called the limiting factor. This means that the cysteine is the most challenging for the body to find and hold onto.

Okay, most of us are not biochemists; so let's try to understand this molecule differently.

Let's start by asking: What does it do? While that requires a longer answer, the following is a short list of what glutathione is required for:

Master Anti-oxidant

- Endogenous – made inside of the cell
- Re-stabilizes itself and all other anti-oxidants
- Deals with six categories of free radicals
- Works inside the cell; in the cell membrane; and outside of the cell.

- (most anti-oxidant can deal with one type of free radical, in one area, and then is lost)

Detoxification
- Major component of Phase II in liver detox
- Major component of all cellular detoxification.

Inflammation
- Major component of healthy inflammation resolution
- Important to leukotriene synthesis (they are important inflammatory mediators).

Hormone regulation
- Involved either directly or indirectly with all hormones in the body.

Cellular Energy
- Cellular energy is provided by the ATP; created by the mitochondria – glutathione is the only known molecule that protects the mitochondria.

Prostaglandin synthesis:
- Required for (vasodilation/constriction of smooth muscles (arteries)
- Aggregation and disaggregation of platelets (required for healing and resolving inflammation)
- Regulate calcium movement
- Control cell growth
- Control hormone regulation
- Regulate inflammatory mediation

NO (Nitric Oxide) regulation, which is important for:

- Hormone regulation
- Vasodilation
- Immune system
- Cellular signaling molecule
- Neural signaling molecule that operates very differently from neurotransmitters.

DNA

- Protects DNA from going sideways; involved in both recontruction or elimination of abnormal DNA
- Also required in protein synthesis

Cellular transport

- Required for most amino acid transportation inside the cells.

Anti-aging

- Involved, like other anti-oxidants, in preventing telomere breakdown but also the only known molecule that can provoke telomere creation.

Calcium movement

- Required for regulation of Calcium movement (gating of cardio cell function).

Respiratory

- 40% required in red blood cells to both pick up/release both O2 and CO2.

Immune System

- Lymphocytes, ie., T cells, B cells, macrophages, TNF, NK, etc, all require about 62% to both develop and function

- Glutathione also regulates balance/ratios in immune cells, i.e., T1 and T2.

Would you believe that most physicians I have talked with over the past few years didn't even know what glutathione was? In addition, I talked to the head of the BioLabs, that do all the blood analysis work, and had to explain glutathione to them!

One can well imagine, that if glutathione is involved in all these different functions in the body, having depleted levels can cause a lot of problems. In fact, some researchers have claimed that there is not a dysfunction, disease, or disorder in the body that is not correlated with low levels of glutathione.

Note, the term correlated. That means that low levels of glutathione did not actually cause the disease. Western science is often misleading in its terminology. A correlational relationship is in no way a causal relationship.

Here's a brief example so that you understand the difference when you are studying, researching, or exploring other medical issues.

If I say, "I always wake up with the sun," that implies a correlational relationship. If I say, "The sun woke me up," that is a causal relationship. I may always wake with the sun because of habit; because I set my alarm clock; because my dogs wake me up; etc. Other factors woke me up but it just happens to correlate with the sunrise.

On the other hand, the sun may wake me up because the sunlight flooded my room. In this case, the sun had a direct causal impact.

When we say that low levels of glutathione are correlated with virtually every disease, disorder or dysfunction in the body, we might be saying:

- The low levels of glutathione caused the disorder.

- Low levels of glutathione created a cascading domino effect that led to the disorder.

- The low levels of glutathione are a result of the disorder.

- Toxins caused low levels of glutathione, which led to an increased accumulation of free radicals, which led to inflammation, which led to the disorder.

- Insufficient nutrients made it difficult to

synthesize glutathione and also contributed to the disorder.

- Toxins turned off the DNA that creates the tools necessary to synthesize glutathione causing a domino effect that lead to the disorder.

- Toxins and other issues used up glutathione faster than the body could make it.

As you can see, when there is a correlational relationship, there can be a lot of different factors involved and various types of causal connections. Okay, we've got the picture so let's move on.

Let's now take a quick look at the different aspects to the glutathione complex that allows it to carry out all of these different functions.

The two most commonly known components of the glutathione complex are the:

- GSH – the reduced state (90%)
- GSSG – the oxidized state (10%)

But other components include:

- GR – glutathione reductase
- Glutathione S transferase (a glutathione enzyme found in cytosol, microsomes and mitochondria)
- Glutathione S-transferase omega 1
- Glutathione peroxidase (a glutathione

enzyme that protects the body reducing lipid hydroperoxides to alcohols and hydrogen peroxide to water)
- S-D-lactoyl-glutathione
- Glutathione synthetase

Are you starting to get an idea of how important glutathione is to the body's functioning? Now here's a brief look at how many ways we can lose glutathione.

- Aging
- Deficient healthy microbiota
- Dehydration
- Drugs (alcohol, tobacco, legal and illegal drugs)
- Exercising past a sweat
- Genetic abnormalities
- Heavy metal toxicity
- Infections
- Inflammatory conditions
- Injuries
- Pesticides and certain food additives
- Pollution
- Poor diet
- Poor sleeping habits
- Radiation
- Stress

- Too much sun
- Toxins

What does this graph mean?

- The horizontal line of the graph indicates the years in your life up to 80 years old.
- The vertical line indicates the amount of glutathione in the system. The units from 0 to 100 are just arbitrary units.
- The blue line indicates how much glutathione we used to lose and how fast.
- The red line indicates how much glutathione we are loosing now and how fast.
- The green line indicates our increasing need for glutathione due to the list of issues identified above.

Oh, dear. That doesn't look too good. But wait. It actually gets worse. One of the things this graph reflects is that about fifty years ago we used to lose

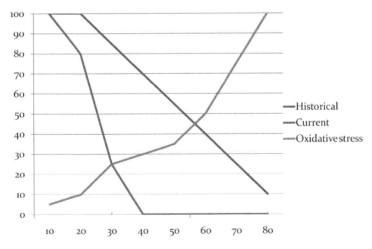

glutathione at a rate of about 1-2% per year from the time we were about twenty years old. Today, we are losing glutathione at a rate of between 12-15% per year and starting at a much younger age.

Now, that really doesn't sound good.

What is good, however, is that we can get the body to start making it again. Oh, thank goodness! We need to make sure the right genes are turned on and that the body has the nutrients to make glutathione – but guess what? We can do that, too. Whew!

Now, let's take a closer look at how glutathione actually functions in the body.

TWO

Glutathione as the Master Anti-oxidant

Glutathione has long been recognized as the Master anti-oxidant. Far more powerful than any supplement, cocktail, or food you can ingest. There is good reason for its reputation.

An anti-oxidant is willing to provide an electron to a free radical in order to stabilize and prevent it from damaging other molecules, although we do have some important free radicals in the body that help a variety of functions, i.e. superoxide dismutase (SOD) and nitric oxide (NO).

Most anti-oxidants can work on one type of free radicals and in a given location. On the surface that sounds good but let's take a closer look.

First off, we have about 10^{12} number of cells in the body and about 10^{32} number of free radicals. That means a 10 with 32 zeroes after it. Get the picture?

Now there are a variety of different types of free radicals:

Oxygen based free radicals aka ROS:

- Hydroxyl radical
- Hydroxyl ion

- Superoxide anion
- Hydrogen peroxide
- Dioxygen O_2

Another group of free radicals are the nitrogen based ones, a.k.a. RNS:

- Peroxynitrite
- Nitrogen dioxide
- Dinitrogen trioxide

And others.

There are also three major locations where different anti-oxidants work:

- In the cells
- In the cell membrane
- Outside of the cells

Different anti-oxidants work on different types of free radicals, and in different locations.

Glutathione, however, works on all types of free radicals in *all* locations. But that isn't all. Most anti-oxidants give away an electron and now they become a free radical. So why do we take them? Well, when our favored anti-oxidants become free radicals, the body has an easier time dealing with them, versus the ones we consider the real bad guys. Again, glutathione takes the cake. Glutathione can re-stabilize itself and thus perform over and over and over again. Not only does it re-stabilize itself, it also re-stabilizes other anti-oxidants, so that they can perform again.

So to summarize:

- Glutathione works on all types of free radicals.
- Glutathione works in all locations.
- Glutathione re-stabilizes itself.
- Glutathione re-stabilizes all other anti-oxidants.

That is a pretty impressive anti-oxidant. This is probably why every cell in the body produces glutathione.

In fact, biologists are claiming that glutathione is a million times more powerful than any other anti-oxidant. The next time you hear advertisements about someone claiming to have found the most powerful anti-oxidant *or* producing the most powerful anti-oxidant combination, you can ask them if they know about what the body produces.

THREE

Glutathione and Detox

You just heard about how effective glutathione is an anti-oxidant but it is just as important in the detoxification mechanisms. Most people associate detoxification with the liver, without realizing that every cell in the body has detox mechanisms. Glutathione is required in every cell to help with those detoxification processes.

This chapter, however, is going to focus on the glutathione that is involved in these detox systems in the liver. It is probably because glutathione plays such a huge part in the liver detox program that we find the highest concentration of glutathione in the liver. So this chapter will focus on glutathione and the liver.

When toxins are fat-soluble molecules, they are difficult to dissolve and eliminate. If they do not get eliminated through the processes in the liver, then the toxins may get stored in the fatty tissues and cell membranes. If the toxins get stored in the fatty tissues, they can stay there for years. If released at a later time due to stress, exercise and fasting, then they can cause symptoms like: stomach pains, nausea, fatigue, poor memory and heart palpitations.

Substances that will provoke Phase I detoxification include:

- Drugs
    - Alcohol
    - Nicotine (in cigarette smoke)
    - Phenobarbital
    - Sulfonamides
    - Steroids
- Environmental toxins
    - carbon tetrachloride
    - exhaust fumes
    - paint fumes
    - dioxin
    - pesticides
- Foods
    - Broccoli
    - Brussels sprouts
    - Cabbage
    - Charcoal-broiled meats
    - High protein diets
    - Oranges
    - Tangerines
- Herbs
    - Caraway seeds
    - Dill
- Nutrients

o Vitamin B1
o Vitamin B3: Niacin
o Vitamin C

If we have a good healthy liver then these toxic molecules go through the two phases of detox in the liver. The first phase involves the P-450 cytochrome system and the toxins are reduced to smaller fragments. This process can actually create even more toxic by-products through the various chemical reactions like oxidation, reduction or hydrolysis.

The second phase involves binding the original molecule to another molecule, which is usually glutathione but may also be glycine or sulfate. This makes the molecule less harmful and water-soluble so that it can be eliminated through the urinary channel or through the bile and stool channel.

There are actually six different Phase II detoxification pathways:

- Glutathione
- Sulfation (the weakest one)
- Methylation (requires glutathione)
- Acetylation
- Glucuronidation
- Amino acids (glycine, taurine, glutamine, arginine, and ornithine).

Consequently, glutathione is not only the most required end component of Phase II detox but it is also required to clean up the toxic mess created by Phase I.

If there isn't sufficient glutathione, to:

- bind with the original toxin in Phase II
- or to eliminate the toxic free radicals
- we end up accumulating toxins in the liver.

Thus, glutathione becomes hugely important to all aspects of the detoxification process.

This liver, the largest organ inside the body, is responsible for over 500 functions and supports all other systems and functions in the body. When the liver is healthy, it is said to clear about 99% of the bacteria and various toxins on the first go around the blood passes through it. So it is vitally important that our liver remains healthy.

Today's statistics, however, are showing that a significant proportion of people have a non-alcoholic fatty liver disorder or otherwise toxic liver by the time they are thirty years old. Oh, oh.

Remember, we already recognized that people are losing between 12%-15% of their glutathione per year from a young age. This will certainly contribute to a dysfunctional liver.

If there is an imbalance between Phase I and Phase II detoxification, due to either a large amount of toxins *or* if exposed to toxins for a prolonged period of time, and if there is insufficient glutathione to take care of the by-products and/or Phase II detox, then a wide variety of possible symptoms may occur as the liver starts to shut down.

A possible short list may include:

- Intolerance to environmental chemicals
- Intolerance to caffeine
- Intolerance to perfumes
- Intolerance to drugs
- Increased risk of liver disease
- Increased risk for a variety of cancers
- Chronic fatigue
- Fibromyalgia

Another aspect to this process is that grapefruit juice actually slows down the Phase I enzyme activity by decreasing the cytochrome P450 activity by about 30%. This can have a number of effects. For instance, it will slow down the elimination of various drugs from the blood. Consequently, you can become toxic on various medications. Note, even acetaminophen can be toxic, if glutathione levels are low.

An alternative way of looking at this is to use grapefruit juice to decrease the amount of drugs you have to take. So, by eating or drinking grapefruit, we increase P450, we lengthen the time a given drug is in the system and thus we need less medication. However, if you chose to do this, you have to monitor the blood rates of the drugs carefully, in order to get the right balance between grapefruit and the drug – otherwise you can become either toxic or depleted. Make sure if you chose this, you do so under the guidance of an informed health practitioner.

FOUR

Glutathione as a Chelator

Chelation is the process of binding ions to heavy metal toxins in the blood to extract them from the blood.

Heavy metal toxicity is a huge issue in today's society. Toxic metals are metals that are poisonous soluble compounds that have no biological role. They can be: non essential minerals or they are not bio-available or they are in forms that are toxic to the body.

Different substances may have different structures, i.e. magnesium has twelve different forms but only three forms are bio-available. You need to know whether your body has the capacity to metabolize and absorb the kind of magnesium you are supplementing with. How do you find out which kind is most applicable for you - go to a good health practitioner who knows what they are doing.

On the other hand, research shows that magnesium stearate, a lubricant compound that is utilized to protect the machinery making the capsules, reduces absorption of whatever compound it is involved in.

But let's look at some of the metal concerns:

The most common heavy metal toxins are:

- Aluminum
- Arsenic
- Cadmium
- Lead
- Mercury

Historically, it was said that you can be more vulnerable to toxins because:

- Genetic predispositions
- Chronic conditions

But today, it is recognized that you can be more vulnerable to these toxins because you have low levels of glutathione.

It can be difficult to eliminate the toxins:

- Due to genetic predispositions (i.e., APO-E 4/3 and 4/4 genotypes are more susceptible to metal toxicities, like mercury).
- If you have chronic health conditions – most people do without even being aware of it due to:
  - Nutrient deficiency
  - Microbiota deficiency
  - Anti-oxidant deficiency
  - Phyto nutrient deficiency. Most people are becoming aware that they require vitamins, minerals, Omega 3 fatty acids and anti-oxidants but they

are not generally aware that we also need the following groups of phytonutrients. Now you are not expected to know these categories or where to find them – but just take a look and get a feeling for what our bodies require:

- Phenolic compounds
    - Natural monophenols
    - Polyphenols
        - Flavonoids
        - Isoflavonoids
        - Flavonolignans
        - Lignans
        - Stilbenoids
        - Curcuminoids
        - Hydrolyzable tannins
    - Aromatic acids
        - Phenolic acids
        - Hydrolycinnamic acids
    - Capsaicin
    - Tyrosol esters
    - Alkylresorcinols
- Terpenes (isoprenoids)
    - Carotenoids (tetraterpenoids)
        - Carotenes
        - Xanthopylls
    - Monoterpenes

- Saponins
- Lipids
- Triterpenoids
- Betalains
- Organosulfides
- Indules, glucosinolates: sulfur compounds
- Protein inhibitors
- Other organic acids

Now all of these categories of naturally occurring chemical compounds found in plants, are required in our bodies. Some provide only one type of function; others a multitude of functions. Some only operate in a given area, i.e., the heart or the liver, while others are more systemic and operate throughout the body.

When the body is deficient in any given nutrient, it has to compensate. When the body starts to compensate, problems start to occur. We may have a dysfunctional liver and not know about it for twenty years; or a dysfunctional kidney for ten years and not know about it. Typically, it's when the body is no longer capable of compensating that we start to notice symptoms.

People who accumulate more than one kind of metal toxicity will have an *accumulative compound effect*. When we are unable to eliminate one kind of metal toxicity, we then become prone to an inability to eliminate a variety of toxicities (i.e. synergistic toxicity according to Dr. Boyd Hayley of University of Kentucky). Let's take a quick look at some of the common signs and symptoms of metal toxicity (and then we will look at the more specific metals, further down:

- Anemia
- Arthritis
- Brain fog and dementias
- Brain and liver damage
- Cancer
- Chronic infections
- Chronic malaise (through general discomfort, fatigue and illness)
- Chronic pain (through muscle, tendons and soft tissues)
- Depression
- Developmental issues: ADHD, slow learning, etc.
- Dizziness
- Fibromyalgia
- Fibrocystic breast disease (from caffeine)
- Food allergies
- Gastrointestinal complaints (diarrhea, constipation, bloating, gas, heartburn, indigestion)
- Migraines and/or headaches
- Mood swings, depression, and/or anxiety

- Nervous system malfunctions – burning extremities, numbness, tingling paralysis, and/or an electrifying feeling throughout the body
- Osteoporosis
- PMS
- Visual disturbances

The following is a more specific list of symptoms associated with given toxins:

1. **Arsenic toxicity**
   - Abdominal pain
   - Cutis edema
   - Diarrhea
   - Excessive salivation
   - Eyelid edema
   - Fatigue
   - Garlic odor on breath
   - Headache
   - Increased pigmentation of palms and soles
   - Kidney failure
   - Limb paralysis
   - Mental impairment
   - Mental signs: Apathy, dementia
   - Mottled brown skin
   - Nausea
   - Paresthesia
   - Paralysis

- Perforation of nasal septum
- Progressive blindness
- Vertigo

2. **Lead toxicity**
   - Abdominal pain
   - Adrenal fatigue/insufficiency
   - Chronic renal failure
   - Cognitive dysfunction
   - Constipation
   - Convulsion
   - Fatigue
   - Gastrointestinal complaints
   - Gout
   - Headache
   - Hemolytic anemia
   - Hypertension
   - Hypothyroid
   - Impotence
   - Irritability
   - Loss of libido
   - Mental symptoms such as anxiety, cognitive dysfunctions, confusions, delusions, depression, disturbing dreams, excitement, restlessness
   - Nausea
   - Peripheral neuropathy
   - Weight loss

3. **Mercury toxicity**
   - Excess salivation
   - Gingivitis
   - Mental symptoms: anorexia, apathy and depression, irritability, mental deterioration, psychosis, shyness Metallic taste in mouth
   - Stomach and Kidney problems
   - Tremors[1]

4. **Copper toxicity**
   - Copper toxicity is a huge factor in the higher incidence of autism in children as well as ADD (attention deficit disorder), teen depression, bipolar disorder, and even schizophrenia.

So if metal toxicity is such a big thing – how do we get it? Here are a few examples:

1. **Acute exposure**
   - Vaccinations that contain thimerosal (mercury preservative)
   - Mishandled metals at the job site
   - Chemical and heavy metal spills

2. **Chronic exposure**
   - Food: fish with mercury, chicken with arsenic; etc.
   - Water: Tap or bottled
   - Air

- Household cleaning products
- Personal hygiene products
  o Makeup
  o Skin whitening products that contain mercury (11) chloride
  o Anti-per spirants with aluminum
- Household issues
  o Florescent lamps
  o Living in a home with paints older than 1978
  o Smoking and/or inhaling second hand smoke
  o Fillings/amalgams, not just mercury but numerous toxic metals
  o Drugs and vaccinations
- Environmental issues
  o Living near a landfill
  o Working in an environment where exposure is prevalent (i.e. dentist's office).

So now we are getting the picture. We are overloaded with heavy metal toxins; our body is not making the necessary glutathione to chelate them – so what do we do?

Historically, the following nutrients were utilized to diminish metal toxicity:

1. **Vitamins**
- Vitamin C

2. Specific molecules
- Alpha lipoic acid (ALA)
- Bioflavonoids
- CoQ10
- L-cysteine
- L-methionine
- NAC – N-Acetyl-Cysteine

3. Botanicals
- Cilantro
- Ginkgo biloba
- Hawthorne berry
- Kale
- Pinus maritima (OPC)

By far the most potent is glutathione. In fact, in treating many blood toxicities glutathione will be injected right into the blood. The challenge with this procedure is that the feedback loops in the cells say, "Okay, we have enough glutathione," and stop making any more. So that might be the residual side effect.

So, again we come back to:

1. Making sure our genes are turned on to make the mRNA tools that make glutathione.
2. Making sure we have the nutrients to support all the different components of the glutathione complex.

That is only one piece of the toxicity issue. There are all kinds of toxicities beside heavy metal toxicity. Let's look some more.

There is a wide variety of toxins that we put into our bodies from all the same sources: air, water, food, personal hygiene, household cleaning products, pharmaceutical drugs and vaccinations, and our environment.

These toxins include:
- POPs – Persistant organic pollutants
- PCBS – includes insecticides, herbicides, pesticides, etc
- Colourants, stabilizers, preservatives

With all that going on, how can you help your liver? You can work with various foods, vitamins, minerals, and phytonutrients.

For instance, the following foods help to support liver detoxification:
- Cabbage family
- Cold-water fish
- Flaxseed oil, hemp seed, salba/chia seed
- Fruits (fresh)
- Garlic, Onions – same family
- Nuts and seeds
- Oils: Safflower, sesame seed, sunflower seed, walnut, wheat germ
- Vegetables (fresh)

And we can provide the following nutritional supplements:

- Bioflavonoids
- Black currant seed oil
- Borage oil
- Carotenes
- Coenzyme Q10
- Copper
- Evening primrose oil
- Iron
- Lecithin
- Magnesium
- Manganese
- N-acetyl-cysteine (stabilizes cysteine to help synthesize glutathione)
- Selenium
- Silymarin (milk thistle) – not a detoxifier as once believed; it provokes the liver to renew itself, thus helping to eliminate the toxins in the process
- Trace minerals
- Vitamin A
- Vitamin Bs: B2 (riboflavin), B3 (Niacin), B6 (pyridoxine), B9 (Folic acid), B12
- Vitamin C (not laboratory ascorbic acid)
- Vitamins D, E, K
- Zinc

We *can* turn on the DNA that makes the mRNA tools that synthesize glutathione *and* we can provide the nutrients that support the glutathione complex.

See Appendix for further information.

FIVE

Glutathione and the Mitochondria

You now have a bit of an understanding of:

- How complex and inter-dynamic our bodies are.
- How many compounds are bodies are required to make by day, hour, second.
- How many nutrients our body requires.
- How many ways we might get toxic.
- How many ways we need glutathione.
- How many ways we lose this precious glutathione.
- How many metals we need to chelate with glutathione.

Don't worry – you are not going to get tested on all this. Whew!

Now, let's look at one of the cells' organs. Organs in a cell are called organelles. One of them is called the mitochondria.

Some believe that at one time the mitochondria functioned on their own. In today's world, the mitochondria are inter-dependent with us. We cannot live without them and they cannot live without us. That's nice – but what do they do?

Amongst other functions, mitochondria are probably the most well known for their double membrane that embodies the ETC or electron transfer chain. This chain consists of twenty-two movements that ultimately provide the ATP, a.k.a. adenosine triphosphate, a.k.a. the fuel for those thousands of enzymes that the body makes.

Now remember, whether the body is breaking something down (food particles or a compound that is no longer needed), building something up (collagens, enzymes, hormones, neurotransmitters, etc.), transforming one compound into another (recycling neurotransmitters, making amino acids, eliminating toxins, etc.) enzymes are required. Enzymes require fuel to function. Most enzymes require the mitochondria's ATP/fuel to function.

Here is a quick look at the importance of these mitochondria. Each cell will contain as many mitochondria as it requires to produce enough ATP to support the necessary fuel needs of that given cell.

Consequently, a heart cell, for example, will contain anywhere between 1000–2500 mitochondria to produce enough fuel to keep that heart functioning 24/7. The only time the heart should stop beating is when you sneeze. I'll bet you didn't know that.

Different cells have different numbers of mitochondria – you get that – but what in the body, or the cell, protects that mitochondria so that it keeps functioning and keeps producing fuel? You guessed it – glutathione.

This shows you another reason every cell in the body requires glutathione and another reason you need to protect it.

By the way, Chronic Fatigue Syndrome is thought to be the result of two inter-related issues: Low glutathione and poor mitochondrial functioning.

SIX

Glutathione and the Telomeres

Telomeres? Oh no, not something else to learn!

As with the explanation of mitochondria, we are going to have another simple quick chapter to explain telomeres.

Note, the length of the chapter does *not* correlate with the importance of the topic. But rather, in an attempt to make this easy, I am only presenting the information that is easier to understand. Again, you are not going to get tested on this information.

What exactly are these telomeres? Telomeres are a collection of about 1500 units of nucleotides found at the ends of the chromosomes on the DNA strands – remember you have DNA in each cell – with 23 pairs of chromosomes and some 25,000 genes.

Telomeres protect the chromosomal information in the DNA so that all the information gets replicated. With each replication, however, we lose telomeres. Further, free radicals and other compounds can destroy telomeres.

Research now indicates, although it is an old theory, that when the telomeres get too short, the cell cannot replicate and is thus one of the causes of old age, cancer and other dysfunctions.

So what role does glutathione play? Glutathione not only protects the telomere units *but* it also provokes the telomerase enzyme that is required to make new telomere units. Yeah, glutathione!

We know that glutathione protects the body from aging by:

1. Both protecting the old and provoking the synthesis of new telomere units
2. Protecting the mitochondria that makes the fuel that supports any metabolic process
3. Chelating the metals out of the blood
4. Detoxing the cells and the liver
5. Providing the best anti-oxidant to free radicals.

Not bad, for one little compound. What is even better – it did all of this for you – without your even knowing it was there or what it did. Wow!

Probably, if you are like most people, you just keep eating and drinking toxic foods, breathing toxic air, smothering your body with toxins, cleaning your house with toxins, etc. Have you ever considered how abusive you are to your body and to that poor little glutathione compound?

When you go to the MD, you just add to the problem with the artificial, toxic compounds he or she prescribes. These compounds, known as drugs, further deplete the body of nutrients and make the glutathione work even harder. Oh, dear...

SEVEN

Glutathione and DNA protection

As we have seen, glutathione is involved in a lot of different functions. It is hard to say which is the most important. The challenge is that, as we noted in Chapter 1, all the functions are inter-dependent throughout the whole body. Let's focus on the DNA here.

There are a variety of DNA processes that glutathione is involved in:

- DNA synthesis (or manufacturing)
- Protects proteins for gene transcription during cell cycle progression (coping of the DNA for the formation of a new cell)
- Regulates posttranslational systems and metabolic proteins (the step in protein synthesis whereby amino acids are used to create proteins OR other biofunctional groups are added to amino acids: lipids, carbs, acetates, phosphates, etc)
- DNA repairs are dependent on glutathione
- Redox regulation (movement of electrons)
- Signaling pathways
- Protects DNA from damage[1]

So what does all that mean? It means that there are many ways that DNA can go sideways and a variety of ways that glutathione can either correct the DNA or eliminate the new dysfunctional cell.

When abnormal or damaged DNA is allowed to replicate itself, it provides one of the many possible causes of cancer. Thus, we need very tight control over the replication process. While glutathione is only one of several compounds that are involved in this process, what makes glutathione stand out is the number of roles it plays.

EIGHT

Glutathione and the Respiratory System

What does glutathione have to do with the respiratory system? Do you know what RBCs are?

Your blood is made up of RBCs (red blood cells) and WBCs (white blood cells). Although both originate in the bones, the red blood cells are considered to be part of your respiratory system, while the white blood cells are considered a part of the immune system.

Remember from the fun facts in Chapter 1, that you make about 250–300 million red blood cells a second. You have about 250 trillion red blood cells in your body and every one of those red blood cells requires glutathione – that's a lot of glutathione.

Red blood cells go through the lungs and pick up oxygen and drop off C02 in the alveoli (you have millions of alveoli in each lung). The blood then goes back through the heart and out into the body. A unit of blood will travel through the body three times in a minute, delivering oxygen and collecting C02.

Both the red blood cells and the alveoli require glutathione. As usual, the glutathione provides both the detox and anti-oxidant functions and in the process, but it also provides some other functions.

One function that the glutathione provides is to protect the RBC scavenging (free radical and chemokine) function.[1]

The anti-oxidant function of glutathione in red blood cells also protects the red blood cells against *Heinz bodies.* Heinz bodies are damaged hemoglobin components. Usually the damage is due to oxidative stress but it can also be caused by inherited mutations. Damaged red blood cells are normally cleared out in the spleen by macrophages. If too many cells are damaged, this can lead to Heinz body anemia. (anemia is a decrease in the number of red blood cells; commonly caused by low iron or low Vitamin B12; but also caused by a variety of other issues as well).

Heinz bodies can also be found with chronic liver disease – the correlation is obvious when you consider that low glutathione levels lead to a toxic liver.

Glutathione also enhances the intracellular magnesium allowing the red blood cells to function more effectively. [2]

One interesting piece of information here is that researchers found that alcohol abuse, even before liver cirrhosis occurs, can deplete the alveoli (where the red blood cells exchange CO_2 for oxygen) by

80%. The alveoli then allow fluid in and the exchange can no longer take place.[3]

Specific disorders related to the lungs and low levels of glutathione include:

- Asthma
- ARDS aka acute respiratory distress syndrome
- COPD aka chronic obstructive pulmonary disease (bronchitis and emphysema)
- Cystic Fibrosis
- Lung Injury

So we need to get those glutathione levels up for our lungs as well.

NINE

Glutathione and the Immune System

First off, just as a side note, you might be interested in knowing that about 90% of your immune system resides in your gut! And, immune issues in your gut can cause issues throughout the body. Therefore, we have lots of good reasons to take care of our gut.

The immune system is made up of two predominant components called the Innate System (the immune cells innately know what to do) and the Adaptive Immune System (the immune cells learn along the way, in reaction to the environment).

One group of immune cells are called the leukocytes or white blood cells. There are about 7000 white cells per microliter of blood.

The leukocytes include the following types of cells: basophil, eosinophil, lymphocyte, monocytes and neutrophils.

They also require glutathione. I bet you already knew that.

Glutathione is crucial to the immune system in a number of ways:

- It actually promotes the synthesis of white blood cells.
- Studies show that increasing levels of glutathione results in the proliferation (increased numbers) of lymphocytes AND the differentiation or specialization of lymphocytes into natural killer cells (NK) and T cells.[1]
- It is important to regulate the ratios of certain types of white blood cells.
- If either Th1 (the type of cell that is in the first line of defense; or which drives cellular immunity or cell mediated immunity: used for viruses, bacteria) or Th2 (which drives the humeral (learned) immunity: and fights against bacteria, toxins, allergens found in the blood and other body fluids) is dominant then various other diseases will occur. It is currently believed that the balance between Th1 and Th2 can shift for a variety of reasons but will typically come back into balance. The problem is when this balance is not regained.
- For instance, if Th1 is dominant, the following may occur:
  - Celiac disease
  - Chronic viral infections
  - Crohn's Disease
  - Grave's Disease
  - Hashimoto's thyroiditis

- Lichen planus
- Multiple Sclerosis
- Psoriasis
- Rheumatoid arthritis
- Sjogren's syndrome
- Type 1 diabetes.

If Th2 is dominant than the following might occur:

- Allergic dermatitis
- Allergies
- Asthma
- Atopic eczema
- Cancer
- Inflammatory Bowel disease
- Lupus
- Multiple chemical sensitivity
- Scleroderma
- Sinusitis
- Ulcerative Colitis.[2]

Note: there is still some controversy over this. [3]

However, glutathione protects the white blood cells, prior to, during, and after activation.[4]

While glutathione benefits the immune system, there is another important side benefit. Remember, about 90% of the immune system is in the gut. A big interactive part of the immune system is the microbiota. When glutathione supports the immune system, it is actually helping to support the microbiota, which in turn helps to support the immune system. What teamwork! They should get an Olympic gold metal!

Microbiota are the current hot topic in physiological sciences. It is no longer accepted that they play a minor role in our overall health but rather a huge inter-dynamic role.

Science is even now exploring whether the microbiota can change our DNA. Certainly there are more microbiota DNA in our gut than our combined cellular DNA throughout the cells in our body. We know that different species can change their DNA utilizing the host. Now we may find that the type, ratios, volumes of different microbiota can actually change our DNA.

In consideration that research is now revealing that the microbiota in your gut can have an impact on:

- Depression
- Bipolar
- Schizophrenia
- Parkinson's
- Alzheimer's
- High blood pressure
- Obesity
- Diabetes
- Liver health
- And more…

It is wise to take care of those good bacteria.

For the purpose of this book, research is currently struggling to understand whether microbiota produce glutathione for us, for the gut, or just for themselves. Regardless of the answer, they require glutathione as well.

TEN

Glutathione and the Gastro Intestinal System

As much as we require all kinds of nutrients from the food we eat, food is also loaded with all kinds of things from which we need to protect ourselves. The mucosal tract is where the predominance of our immune system resides. The mucosal membrane is not only lined with various types of cells from the immune system and the microbiota but also with glutathione. The highest concentration is found in the duodenum.

In addition, various foods are loaded with glutathione, which contribute to the amounts of glutathione found there. However, the majority of glutathione will be broken down into the three amino acids by the hydrochloric acid in the stomach.

Other factors contributing to the levels of glutathione found in the duodenum include: the total level of glutathione throughout the body; the amount of toxins in the body, pharmaceutical drugs consumed, drugs and alcohol consumed, and the age of the individual.

Research has found that there is a direct inverse correlation between the levels of glutathione found in the intestines and the amount of damage to the mucosal membrane. That means, that as the levels of glutathione go down, the amount of damage goes up.

The glutathione found in the duodenum has a variety of roles:

- anti-oxidant
- elimination of toxins
- regulation of inflammation
- stimulate synthesis and reaction of the immune system cells.

Gastrointestinal glutathione peroxidase is thought to prevent the absorption of hydroperoxides.

Research also suggests that gastrointestinal glutathione is also involved in cell growth and differentiation. [1]

Foods that contain high levels of glutathione that can benefit your gastrointestinal tract are:

- Asparagus
- Avocados
- Raw goat milk
- Walnuts

Remember, however, that the glutathione in these foods is usually broken down in the hydrochloric acid. In the duodenum, the cells still have access to all of the amino acids (including the unstable cysteine) so that the cells can easily make the required glutathione they require.

ELEVEN

Glutathione and the Inflammatory System

There are a variety of ways that glutathione interacts with the inflammatory system:

1. The inflammatory system is part of the immune system and we have already explored how glutathione impacts the immune system.
2. Glutathione chelates heavy metal toxins, which create inflammation.
3. Glutathione provides the anti-oxidant for free radicals that can provoke inflammation.
4. Glutathione detoxes toxins that provoke inflammation.
5. The most direct way that glutathione interacts with the inflammatory system is by impacting the synthesis of leukotrienes. Leukotrienes are a family of inflammatory mediators produced in leukocytes and other immune cells. When glutathione is depleted, the body stops making leukotriens.[1]

Similarly, levels of glutathione are directly related to the amount of prostaglandins synthesized.[2] In addition to regulating inflammatory mediation, prostaglandins are also involved in the following processes:

- Both constriction and vasodilation of the smooth muscles in the arteries
- Both aggregation and disaggregation of platelets
- Induce labor
- Sensitize spinal neurons to pain
- Regulate calcium movement
- Regulate hormones
- Control cell growth
- Decrease intraocular pressure
- Thermoregulatory processes in the hypothalamus to produce fever
- Inhibit hydrochloric acid secretion in the stomach walls[3.]

Again, the research shows that: either by the total amounts (concentrations of) or by the ratios of different components of glutathione; glutathione determines whether the body will synthesize a variety of compounds that regulate not only inflammation but also a wide variety of other functions.

So now, consider all the different diseases, disorders and dysfunctions that are either caused by or result in inflammation – that is almost all of them.

In fact, many will argue that inflammation is the cause of virtually all disorders, diseases and dysfunctions in the body.

So when we move a step back from the inflammation, and understand the role that glutathione plays in inflammation; we can understand why glutathione researchers say that depleted glutathione is behind the excessive inflammation.

Now, let's take it one step further and look at the variety of situations that can cause inflammation. These include:

- excess free radicals
- excess toxins
- excess metal toxicity
- insufficient immune system regulators
- insufficient inflammatory mediators/regulators.

And what have we discovered is the one common denominator behind all of these issues? Of course, it's glutathione.

TWELVE

Glutathione and the Cardiovascular System

Glutathione is also an important component in the cardiovascular system. You already know of a few of the reasons:

1. Red blood cells and the delivery of oxygen and the elimination of C02.
2. Inflammatory conditions – inflammation in the vascular system, *not* cholesterol, is the real culprit – which alternative medicine has claimed for eons now. Finally, conventional medicine is catching up. In fact, cholesterol has been identified as the firefighter at the fire, whereas inflammation is causing the fire.
3. And you know now of a host of contributing factors that cause inflammation.

There are huge numbers of resources identifying the cholesterol myth from researchers like Dr. Ravnskov, MD, PhD, from the book called *The Cholesterol Myth*, to sites like Dr. Mercola[1], or Dr. Sears[2] or Dr. Hyman, to news broadcasts like BBC[3], or youtube[5,6] to scientists such as Dr. Lindell.[7]

Cholesterol becomes a problem when it is oxidized and, of course, we know that with sufficient glutathione this doesn't happen because it is glutathione is the master anti-oxidant that prevents the oxidation.

Like so many health issues, conventional medicine is misguided. Why is that?

1. The pharmaceutical companies are responsible for most of the medical curricula in North America.
2. They are responsible for the protocol and procedure manuals that the physicians are taught to abide by.
3. They provide the programs for continuing education for the physicians.
4. They control what medical journals are allowed to publish.

Physicians who are truly objective and recognize that the body requires good healthy nutrients in order to function, as we outlined in Chapter 1, represent the few who are:

1. Taking more training
2. Doing their research
3. And for the past 10 or more years have labelled their new emerging field as "Functional Medicine"

However, let's get back to glutathione and the cardiovascular system. Western medicine is slowly catching up and realizing that inflammation and oxidative stress (the result of excessive amounts of free radicals) are the causes of cardiovascular disease.

1. Reducing the amount of free radicals or oxidative stress in the body in turn reduces inflammation.
2. Reducing heavy metal toxicity, in turn reduces inflammation.
3. Reducing toxicity, in turn reduces inflammation.

Reducing any of the three above will result in lower levels of damaged or weakened blood vessels, which in turn can cause inflammation. Now you may have noted two things here:

1. The common denominator is inflammation – not cholesterol.
2. Glutathione eliminates all the precursors to inflammation.

So I guess we need to get our glutathione levels up!

Another problem that can cause cardiovascular issues is thrombosis, or blood clots. Do you remember in the previous chapter, we discussed how glutathione regulates platelets, the components in the blood that orchestrate clotting? Incredible isn't it? No matter which turn we make, we come back to glutathione…

But let's not stop there. Another common cardiovascular issue is high blood pressure. Any issue that causes inflammation in the arteries and/or restricts the blood flow is going to cause high blood pressure. So, of course there is a natural correlation between low levels of glutathione and high blood pressure.

But there are also other issues that cause high blood pressure, too. Let's take a look.

- The arteries not expanding and contracting properly – glutathione regulates the control of nitric oxide and prostaglandins – both involved in the vasodilation/vasoconstriction of the arteries.
- The kidneys not filtering the blood properly – go to Chapter 16.
- The liver not detoxing the blood properly – go to Chapter 3.
- The adrenals pumping out too much adrenaline – go to Chapter 13.

All issues actually come back to glutathione.
So to conclude, increasing glutathione will:

- Lower blood pressure
- Decrease inflammation
- Improve vascular health
- Improve immune function
- Protect against free radicals and oxidative stress

- Protect other anti-oxidants so that they can do the multitude of other things that they might also be capable of doing
- Regulate inflammatory mediators
- Regulate platelets to provide enough clotting without too much
- Remove heavy metals and other toxins that harm the vascular lining
- Ultimately reduce cardiovascular disease, heart attacks and strokes.

And the gold medal goes to: Glutathione.

THIRTEEN

Glutathione and the Neurological System

In consideration of the fact that I practiced as a psychologist for over twenty years *before* becoming a Doctor of Natural Medicine and acquiring training in the string of other modalities I accrued, I love this particular chapter.

For similar reasons that glutathione has such a big impact on the heart and cardio functioning, glutathione also protects the brain and neural functioning.

Let's take a look at what makes up the brain:

- About 60-70% fats (structure, transports, insulation, energy, etc.)
- Glial cells (both the macroglia and microglia form the maintenance crew of the brain; actually assist the neurotransmitters to make neural connections; and effect various physiological processes like breathing.)
- Neurons (I love this one because you can find statistics that claim you have anywhere between 15-120 billion neurons which form the gray matter. So will the real number please stand up?)

- Neurotransmitters (over 60 different ones)
- Hormones
- Enzymes
- Blood brain barrier (BBB)
- Blood (100,000 miles of blood vessels; about 20% of the body's blood.)
- Cerebral spinal fluid (CSF)
- Uses about 20% of the body's oxygen
- Uses between 20-30% of the calories you eat
- 75% of the brain is water
- Insulin in the brain helps promote memory.
- *And* the second highest concentration of glutathione in the body *occurs in the brain.*

Before we get to the question of how all of this relates to glutathione, I will first explain why I am no longer a psychologist. Just think of all the items listed above and then explain to me why psychologists are given no courses in nutrition?

One of the first books I wrote was on depression and how much of depression is due to issues in the body and discusses various nutritional deficiencies, deficient glutathione, dysfunctional gastro-intestinal tract, dysfunctional liver, dysfunctional adrenals and other issues.

When the college found out that I was not only studying all of these things, but had a number of other degrees and designations in alternative medicine, they claimed that I was practicing non-evidenced based medicine.

I offered to come in and teach but they didn't want that. The premise that psychologists work on is this: If the MD has not identified a physiological cause, i.e. the much misunderstood hypothyroid – then depression is psychological.

The problem here is that psychologists are basing their assumptions on another group of professionals who again have no training in functional medicine or the nutrients the body requires in order to function effectively.

Consequently, psychologists and psychiatrists are at an even greater disadvantage than the MD.

Now the big question is, what does glutathione have to do with any of this? The answer is that the brain, like any other part of the body, is susceptible to:

- Nutrient deficiency
- Oxidative stress
- Toxicity
- Heavy metal toxicity
- Inflammation.

How many of these issues are related to low or depleted glutathione? You know the answer – all of them.

Just think, if the brain contains about 20% of the body's oxygen, how much more susceptible to oxidative stress do you think it is? You're right, a lot more.

As you can imagine, the glutathione content of the brain is largely dependent on the precursors of glutathione that are available in the brain. Moreover, different types of brain cells prefer different types of extracellular glutathione precursors. Furthermore, some types of glial cells even have a role in the metabolism of glutathione.[1]

Studies are starting to reveal that whether you look at the autopsies of people who suffered such maladies as major depression, bipolar disorder or schizophrenia you consistently find:

- Increased oxidative stress
- Depleted levels of glutathione
- Increased levels of inflammation

After reading what you have in this book, does that surprise you?

So, how do you raise glutathione in the brain? One study indicates that calcitriol, the active metabolite of Vitamin D, may be a catalyst for increasing glutathione levels in the brain.[2] Much research has been devoted to Vitamin D and its impact on :

- about 20% of your DNA
- your immune system
- your cardio system, etc.

and now it is even being shown to be a catalyst for glutathione synthesis in the brain.

Nitric oxide, the vasodilator, also has additional functions in the brain. Research is now revealing that if there is a disruption in the NO pathway, this too can cause brain dysfunctions and dementias. Of course, you already know that glutathione is responsible for regulating nitric oxide.[3]

Think for a minute. You now know that:

- The highest concentration of glutathione is in the liver and the second highest is in the brain.
- The brain is dependent on the liver to:
    o Synthesize a number of compounds that the brain requires
    o Take toxins out of the blood so that they don't cross the blood brain barrier
    o To get oxygen to the brain
    o To get sugars out of the blood – processed sugars are hugely toxic to the brain.
- Glutathione is an:
    o anti-oxidant
    o detoxifier
    o chelator
    o regulates hormones
    o regulates anti-inflammatories

It must, therefore, be pretty important to the brain.[4] If these functions are not kept under tight control in the brain, there is going to be a problem. Just imagine the number of disorders that can result from low glutathione in the brain?

- Alzheimer's
- Parkinson's
- Depression
- Schizophrenia
- Lou Gehrig's
- Multiple Sclerosis
- Sleep disorders

Note that each of these disorders can be caused from a number of different issues in the body. For instance:

- Deficiency in fatty acids
- Deficiency in minerals
- Heavy metal toxicity
- Other toxins
- Deficient microbiota
- Etc.

Regardless of whether glutathione is the originating cause of the problem, or a subsequent cause of the problem it is part of the equation. The following activities require a healthy brain:

- Cognition:

- Memory: short term, long term, projective, rote, procedural, episodic
- Constructive reasoning
- Abstract reasoning
- Critical analysis
- Hypothetical reasoning
- Objective perspective
- Self-awareness
- Decision making
- Strategic thinking
- Emotion:
  - Ability to access emotions
  - Ability to effectively express emotions
  - Ability to let go of emotions
- Behaviour:
  - Act responsibly
  - Act with intent
  - Act with cooperation
  - Act with maturity
- Movement:
  - Coordinated movement
  - Intended movement
  - Fine motor movement
- Sensory processing:
  - Ophthalmoception (Sight)
  - Audioception (Sound)
  - Tactioception (Touch)
  - Gastacoception (Taste)
  - Olfacoception (Smell)

- Proprioception (knowing where you are in time and space)
- Equilibrioception (Balance)
- Thermoception (Temperature)
- Nociception (Touch)

Ultimately, we need to keep our glutathione levels up in order to support a healthy brain.

FOURTEEN

Glutathione and the Kidneys

You know that the kidneys are involved in creating urine by filtering out the blood. So you can categorize them as part of the urinary system. On the other hand, they work in conjunction with the liver to eliminate toxins from the body so is it part of the hepatic/liver system. But because they clean the blood, and work at maintaining the required water/salt balance in the blood, they are also part of the cardiovascular system. You decide where you want to place them.

The kidneys are similar to the liver in that these are the only places where glutathione is excreted from the organ cells.

Long before a person requires dialysis, it is recognized that:

- The GSH-GSSG, or glutathione redox cycle is severely impaired.
- Whole blood levels of glutathione are significantly decreased.[1]

According to researchers, oxidative stress as a result of the imbalance between pro-oxidant and anti-oxidant systems in the body, (i.e. low levels of anti-oxidants like glutathione, superoxide dismutase, catalase, etc.) impacts the immune system. The negative impact on the immune system "largely contributes to immune system deregulation and complications observed in end-stage renal disease."[2]

Like so many diseases, the question becomes, did chronic renal insufficiency create the state of oxidative stress or visa versa?

Were the reduced glutathione levels that allow for the increased oxidative-damaged compounds, that the kidneys had to eliminate, the cause of kidney insufficiency? Or did the progressive kidney failure or dialysis treatment cause impairment to the glutathione process?

Research shows that oxidative stress biomarkers (i.e. markers in the blood that indicate oxidative stress) are already elevated at the early stages of chronic kidney disease, and simply progresses as the kidneys deteriorate.

Why does this happen? One theory is that people with kidney issues have an inability to absorb and/or utilize cysteine. Thus, they are not making glutathione. Some clinical research studies are now looking at providing these clients with cysteine, N-acetyl cysteine or glutathione. So far, the results indicate that as long as they are provided with one of the above, their improvement continues but returns to pre-treatment levels when treatment is discontinued.

Still, taking the supplemental treatment sounds far better than dialysis.

FIFTEEN

Glutathione and the Skeletal System

What does glutathione have to do with the skeletal system? Would you believe skeletal glutathione is connected to estrogen levels?

Research has found that estrogen deficiency leads to glutathione deficiency in bones, which leads to osteoporosis. Whereas increasing glutathione prevented estrogen deficiency bone loss.[1] Catalase, another anti-oxidant, prevented ovariectomy-induced bone loss. [2]

A simpler study, conducted back in 1991 showed that there was a direct correlation between reduced levels of glutathione and reduced bone density. [3]

Let's look at one of the most common skeletal issues: arthritis. Arthritis actually means joint inflammation: arth"" (joint) and "itis" (inflammation). As simple as it sounds, there are over 100 different inflammatory conditions associated with the skeleton. They may involve the bursae (bursitis) or the tendons (tendinitis). They may be localized, like gout, or systemic, like fibromyalgia. Regardless of what the type of problem is, it is associated with pain.

Conditions like rheumatoid arthritis are thought to

be due to an interesting complication, both an overactive and an underactive immune system. Tricky. How does the body do that? Well, it appears that the B cells in the immune system are over-active while the T cells of the immune system are under-active.

So, you don't want to take immune suppressant drugs. You want to balance the immune system. And you already know who is up for the job. Yes, glutathione.

We already know that glutathione is involved in the inflammatory system and we also know that glutathione is involved in the immune system.

Why not just take painkillers or anti-inflammatories? Painkillers and prescription anti-inflammatories don't solve the underlying problem; they simply mask the symptoms until you need to take them again.

In addition, both can actually destroy the glutathione in the liver as the liver metabolizes them. Oh my! We don't want that. Furthermore, the painkillers can actually increase the risk of a heart attack. Double oh, my!

Remember, in addition to glutathione, there are all kinds of foods that are rich in the omega 3 anti-inflammatories.

SIXTEEN

Glutathione and the Muscular System

Sometimes the muscles are included with the skeletal system, i.e. musculoskeletal but here we will deal with them separately.

Working out is important for the muscles. Actually, movement of any kind is important for the muscles. Gyms and trainers will often provide misleading information concerning the importance of various types of cardio, aerobic, weight training, etc. but all you really need is movement.

There are a variety of movements that are very good for the muscles:

- Walking
- Bicycling
- Tai Chi
- Yoga
- Qigong
- Pilates

The challenge with a lot of exercise programs is that they can provoke two things you don't want:

- Depleted glutathione
- Enlarged left ventricle in the heart

When you exercise past a sweat, you deplete glutathione, which slows down the capacity of the muscle to rebuild. Research also shows that subjects with increased levels of glutathione also have leaner muscles over those with depleted levels.[1]

Weightlifters especially, want muscle to break down so that they can build it stronger. Other hard training athletes also require extra glutathione both for *performance* and to *shorten recovery time*. Breaking down muscle tissue results in a massive increase of free radicals and may also release toxins.[2]

We know by now that glutathione is the number one contender in dealing with these issues.

SEVENTEEN

Weight Loss

If glutathione is helpful for everything else, why not weight loss? Let's look at what we already know and see if we can come to some conclusions.

1. Eliminating excess free radicals helps the body to function more effectively – including managing weight better.
2. Eliminating heavy metals and other toxicities, helps the body to function more effectively – including managing weight better.
3. Strengthening the immune system, most of which resides in the gut, helps more effective food metabolism, which helps the body to function more effectively – including managing weight better.
4. Strengthening and protecting the liver helps the body function more effectively – including managing weight better.
5. Supporting and strengthening the cardiovascular system moves more oxygen into the body and more CO_2 out of the body more effectively – including managing weight better.

6. Supporting and strengthening the kidneys allows the body to eliminate wastes more effectively – which helps manage weight better.
7. Strengthening muscles utilizes more calories and allows the body to function more effectively – including managing weight better.

It would appear that having good healthy levels of glutathione would support a weight management program. Although, you will have greater success with a weight management program if you address a wide number of other issues like these:

- Eat a whole food diet with good nutrient base.
- Eliminate unhealthy, nutrient deficient "food" products such as:
  o Artificial foods
  o Microwaved foods
  o Pasteurized foods
  o Fast foods
- Eat a good volume and various types of microbiota (fermented foods).
- Eat foods that create a healthy pH balance (fruits and vegetables).
- Eat foods that provoke a good production of food metabolizing enzymes (ginger & tumeric).

- Eat foods that support a healthy liver to metabolize compounds from the gut (bitter foods are great for the liver).
- Eliminate toxins like:
  - Processed sugars, high fructose foods, artificial sugars
  - AGE (advanced glycation end products) like ice cream, potato chips, French fries, baking.
  - Heavy metals
  - Toxins from:
    - POPs (persistant organic pollutants)
    - PCBs (pesticides, herbicides, insecticides, etc)
    - Colorants, Stabilizers, Preservatives
- Get off pharmaceutical drugs and illegal drugs.
- Look at underlying life themes, value systems and negative self-images that may be contributing to your weight management program.
- Increase your body's movement. The body was designed to move.

Add in increased glutathione production and you have a good healthy plan for any weight management program.

EIGHTEEN

Glutathione and Cancer

Glutathione is important in both the prevention and the treatment of cancer. Why?

If we can reduce excess free radicals, heavy metal toxicity, and other toxins, we are going to reduce our risk of cancer.

But there is another important variable that we need to take a look at – our DNA. When the DNA goes sideways and the body doesn't correct it or eliminate it, we evolve cancer cells, remember Chapter 7?

With regard to cancer itself, glutathione plays both a protective/preventative role and a pathogenic role. As a preventative, we have listed a vast number of functions that glutathione supports, that protect us from cancers, including its capacity to remove and detox carcinogens.

However, certain types of cancers embrace glutathione in order to protect their own cells.[1] For instance, some types of pancreatic cancers have a higher level of glutathione.[2] Glutathione may also protect the turned off apoptosis in some types of colorectal cancers.[3]

On the other hand, glutathione will also turn apoptosis (DNA pre-programmed cell death, which is turned off in cancer cells) back on, in cancer cells.[4]

So, why the conflict? There are various suggested possibilities.

Like all other disorders, cancers have a variety of causes.

1. There may be more types of glutathione than we currently know.
2. There may be other variables involved that we have not yet identified.
3. Could the role of glutathione be altered due to the type of chemotherapy applied? We don't know yet.
4. Is the conflict a variable we don't yet understand in the study or analysis, what the intent of the study is, and who is paying for the study?
5. Many of the anti-cancer drugs will also have opposite roles, i.e. turn apoptosis on and off, increase and decrease proliferation, etc. depending on the type of cell and external stimulus.[5]
6. In consideration of #5, perhaps we need to have a better understanding of what is causing the cancer. Is it internal to a cell? Is it the result of the surrounding environment? Is it due to pH levels, lack of glutathione, the

result of psychological factors as identified in New German Therapy, or something else?

Ultimately, there are too many unanswered questions. If, like the different types of chemotherapy, it can be both a benefit and a deterrent depending on the type of cancer cell and the location of the cancer, well, there are still just too many unknowns.

What we do know is that good healthy levels of glutathione prevent cancer.

NINETEEN

Conclusion

You now have a general idea, on a superficial level, of some of the attributes of glutathione:

- Master anti-oxidant
- Chelator
- Cell and liver detoxifier
- Regulates anti-inflammatory systems
- Regulates nitric oxide
- Required for red blood cells to function
- Required by the immune system: development, regulation, response
- Required to protect the DNA, telomeres and mitochondria
- Required by the cardio, neural system, the kidney system,
- Required for effective functioning in the skeletomuscular system

Geneticists have now identified some of the genes contributing to making the mRNA tools that synthesize glutathione, although these genes are often turned off, or become turned off, early in life.[1]

But we also know that we can turn them back on again.

You know that we need glutathione now more than ever *and* that we are losing it faster than ever.

So how do we increase glutathione in our bodies?

First, we need to make sure the genes to make glutathione are turned on. One way we can do this is with a product called Protandim. Protandim is a five-herb formulation, being studied in over twenty universities. The reason for the large number of studies is the excitement over the fact that Protandim turns on thousands of genes in our 25,000-gene pool.

The studies now show that it turns on the genes associated with:

- Anti-inflammatory pathways
- Anti-fibrosis pathways
- Anti-oxidant pathways:
  - Glutathione
  - Super oxide dismutase
  - Catalase

Of course, the component of interest here is the glutathione. Once we get these genes turned on then we can start supplying the body with the nutrients it needs to make the glutathione.

Now we can do this in different ways:

1. Eat the foods that are rich in the molecules required for just GSH.

2. Eat the foods that are rich in the molecules required for the whole glutathione complex.
3. Take supplements that support the GSH synthesis.
4. Take supplements that support the whole GSH complex.

Lets start with the top of the list. The rate-limiting factor in making glutathione is the amino acid cysteine. An example of rate-limiting would be, if I were to ask you to make pancakes for a 100 people and gave you an unlimited supply of flour, milk and baking powder but only one egg. The one egg would be the rate-limiting factor.

When the body is making glutathione, the rate-limiting factor is cysteine. We tend to lose it very easily so we need to take this into consideration when providing the body with nutrients to make glutathione. There are a number of ways of doing this involving both foods and supplements. Let's look at both:

Foods

1. Cysteine is a sulfur-rich amino acid that is abundant in:

    • Eggs
    • Garlic and onions
    • Whey protein (bioactive and made from undenatured (or nondenatured) proteins = the cysteine is more bioavailable)

2. Cyanohydroxybutene, a plant phytonutrient found in broccoli, cauliflower and cabbage, kale) enhances glutahtione production

3. Green tea, fish oil and resveratrol also house substances that switch on genes responsible for making glutathione

4. We could try eating glutathione rich foods like:

- Asparagus
- Avocado
- Grapefruit
- Melons
- Peaches
- Spinach
- Squash

There is a benefit and a challenge with these foods. Glutathione tends to break down in the hydrochloric acid of the stomach. Even if it doesn't, we don't have the transport mechanisms to get glutathione into the cells.

The upside of this is that it does provide glutathione and its composites for a variety of functions in the gut.

Another point we need to remember with these foods is that any significant heat or any microwaving destroys anti-oxidants. So these are good foods to:

- Eat raw
- Steam
- Cook at very low heats.

Supplements

Taking straight glutathione doesn't work for two reasons. As mentioned earlier, we break it down in the stomach and end up losing the cysteine. Two, even if it stayed together we cannot transport it into the cell. So what can we do?

1. We can take supplements that support the synthesis of glutathione:
   - NAC (N-acetyl-cysteine), which stabilizes the cysteine and allows us to absorb it to utilize in making glutathione.
   - Amino acid supplementation to make sure we get the amino acids.
   - Alpha-lipoic-acid which has been shown to help restore glutathione.
   - Melatonin, which has been shown to stimulate the glutathione enzyme, glutathione peroxidase.
   - Methylation nutrients like Vitamins B6, B9 and B12, which are important in both the production and the recycling of glutathione.
   - Selenium helps the body both produce and recycle glutathione.

- Vitamins C and E work together to recycle glutathione.
- Milk thistle helps boost levels of glutathione.

2. We can take products that claim to have all the nutrients to support glutathione synthesis – either the GSH or the whole complex. I like to use OGF (Original Glutathione Formula by Dr. Keller) to support the nutrients for GSH.

3. We can take supplements that nanosize the glutathione and encapsulated in a phosphor-lipid transport mechanism that crosses the cellular phospholipid membrane. While I am building a client's capacity to make glutathione on their own, I like to use lypo-spheric GSH as it uses a transport mechanism that is made up of 1000mg of essential phospholipids. The body even requires the transport mechanism.[2]

And lo, and behold, even walking or jogging, playing various sports, or strength training for twenty minutes three times a week helps provoke glutathione synthesis.

My company is called Choices Unlimited for Health and Wellness Ltd. The reason for that is because there many ways the body can go out of harmony and balance and any number of healing modalities that can bring the body back into balance. You have choices.

One incredibly effective and useful choice is to bring your glutathione levels up.

Even here, you have a number of choices in how you want to achieve that.

So, in conclusion, here's to:

- ✓ Your choice to embrace a healing journey.
- ✓ Your choice to increase your glutathione levels.
- ✓ Your choice to live life to the fullest.

APPENDIX

We are still waiting for the legal permission papers from those companies that we would like to have listed here.

Until those papers are received you are welcome to contact Dr. Holly for further information:

drholly@choicesunlimited.ca

You can also go to the website:
www.choicesunlimited.ca for further information.

FOOTNOTES

Chapter 4

[1]Santangelo,F, et al. Restoring glutathione as a therapeutic strategy in chronic kidney disease. Found in: http://www.diagnose-me.com/cond/C15891.html

Chapter 7

1 Chatterjee, Anupam.   Reduced Glutathione: A Radioprotector or a Modulator of DNA-Repair Activity? Found in:
http://www.google.com.mx/url?sa=tandrct=jandq=and
esrc=sandfrm=1andsource=webandcd=5andved=0CFYQ
FjAEandurl=http%3A%2F%2Fwww.mdpi.com%2F2072-
6643%2F5%2F2%2F525%2Fpdfandei=VIuHUq_zNoTHiw
Llg4HICgandusg=AFQjCNGGoiHI7NCTbnUiIEtJk73_F0
Jo8g

Chapter 8

[1] Dumaswala, UJ, et al. Glutathione protects chemo-kine scavenging and antioxidative defense functions in RBCs. Found in:

http://www.ncbi.nlm.nih.gov/pubmed/11245604

[2] Barbagall, Mario, et al. Effects of Glutathione on Red Blood Cells Intracellular Magnesium. Found In:
http://hyper.ahajournals.org/content/34/1/76.full

[3] Brown L., et al. "Chronic ethanol ingestion and the risk of acute lung injury: a role for glutathione availability?. Found In:

http://www.alcoholjournal.org/article/S0741-8329(04)00104-1/abstract

Chapter 9

[1] Fidelus, Rk, et al. Modulation of intracellular glutathione concentrations alters lymphocyte activation and proliferation. Found In:

http://www.ncbi.nlm.nih.gov/pubmed/3595735

[2] What is the Role of Th1 and Th2 in Autoimmune Disease? Found In:
http://autoimmunepaleo.wordpress.com/2013/01/21/what-is-the-role-of-th1-and-th2-in-autoimmune-disease/

[3] Kidd, P. Th1/Th2 balance: the hypothesis, its limitations, and implications for health and disease. Found In:

http://www.ncbi.nlm.nih.gov/pubmed/12946237

[4] Bounous, Gustavo, John Molson. The Antioxidant System. Found In:

http://www.getimmunocal.com/IMMTOP/Diseases/Cancer/The%20Antioxidant%20System.pdf

Chapter 10

[1] Florian, S., et al. Cellular and subcellular localization of gastrointestinal glutathione peroxidase in normal and malignant human intestinal tissue. Found in:

http://www.ncbi.nlm.nih.gov/pubmed/11811519

Chapter 11

[1] Rouzer, C.A., et al. Depletion of glutathione selectively inhibits synthesis of leukotriene C by macrophages. Found in:
http://www.ncbi.nlm.nih.gov/pmc/articles/PMC319382/

[2] Buckley, BJ, et al. Regulation of endothelial cell prostaglandin synthesis by glutathione. Found In:
http://www.ncbi.nlm.nih.gov/pubmed/1885596

[3] Prostaglandin. Found in:
http://en.wikipedia.org/wiki/Prostaglandin

Chapter 12

[1] Mercola, Joseph. The Cholesterol Myth That Is Harming Your Health. Found In:
http://articles.mercola.com/sites/articles/archive/2010/08/10/making-sense-of-your-cholesterol-numbers.aspx

[2] Sears, Barry. Another new wrinkle in the cholesterol story. Found in:
http://zonediet.com/blog/2011/06/another-new-wrinkle-in-the-cholesterol-story/

3 Hyman, Mark, MD. Glutathione: the mother of all antioxidants. Found in:
http://www.huffingtonpost.com/dr-mark-hyman/glutathione-the-mother-of_b_530494.html

4 BBC: Malhotra, A. Saturated fat heart disease "myth".
http://www.bbc.co.uk/news/health-24625808

5 YOUTUBE: Harvard Profession Reveals the Truth about the Cholesterol Myth. Found in:
http://www.youtube.com/watch?v=iyB5Ylaf_w8

6 Dr. Johnny Bowden "The Great Cholesterol Myth" Found in:
http://www.youtube.com/watch?v=YGOpjPNtjes

7 Lundell, Dwight. Dr. Dwight Lundell on taking statins. Found in: http://www.realfarmacy.com/world-renown-heart-surgeon-speaks-out-on-what-really-causes-heart-disease/

8 Blankenber, Stefan, et al. Glutathione Peroxidase 1 Activity and Cardiovascular Events in Patients with Coronary Artery Disease Found in:
http://www.nejm.org/doi/full/10.1056/NEJMoa030535

Chapter 13

1 Dringen, R. Metabolism and functions of glutathione in brain. Found in:
http://www.ncbi.nlm.nih.gov/pubmed/10880854

2 Garcion, E, New clues about vitamin D functions in the nervous system. Found In:
http://www.ncbi.nlm.nih.gov/pubmed/11893522

[3] Steinert, JR., et al. Nitric oxide signaling in brain function, dysfunction, and dementia. Found in: http://www.ncbi.nlm.nih.gov/pubmed/20817920

[4] Dringen, Ralf. Metabolism and functions of glutathione in brain. Found in: http://members.shaw.ca/duncancrow/GSH-metabolism-in-brain.pdf

Chapter 14

[1] Santangelo, Francesco, et al. Restoring glutathione as a therapeutic strategy in chronic kidney disease. Found in: http://ndt.oxfordjournals.org/content/19/8/1951.full

Chapter 15

[1] Lean, JM, et al. 'Normal skeletal development and regulation of bone formation and resorption'. Found in: http://www.uptodate.com/contents/normal-skeletal-development-and-regulation-of-bone-formation-and-resorption/abstract/100

[2] Lean, JM, et al. 'Normal skeletal development and regulation of bone formation and resorption' Found in: http://www.uptodate.com/contents/normal-skeletal-development-and-regulation-of-bone-formation-and-resorption/abstract/96

[3] Avitabile, M, et al. Correlation between serum glutathione reductases and bone densitometry values. Found in: http://www.ncbi.nlm.nih.gov/pubmed/1821134

Chapter 16

[1] Lifesaving Glutathione. Found In: http://hwifc.com/glutathione/

[2] US Vitamin Injections Explains Glutathione Benefits in Brand New Article. Found In: http://www.prnewswire.com/news-releases/us-vitamin-injections-explains-glutathione-benefits-in-brand-new-article-187449691.html

Chapter 18

[1] Balendiran, GK. The role of glutathione in cancer. Found In: http://www.ncbi.nlm.nih.gov/pubmed/15386533

[2] Schnelldorfer, T. et al. Glutathione depletion causes cell growth inhibition and enhanced apoptosis in pancreatic cancer cells. Found in: http://www.ncbi.nlm.nih.gov/pubmed/11013356

[3] Sidler, D., et al. Thiazolide-induced apoptosis in colorectal cancer cells is mediated via the Jun kinase–Bim axis and reveals glutathione-S-transferase P1 as Achilles' heel. Found in: http://www.nature.com/onc/journal/v31/n37/abs/onc2011575a.html

[4] Donnerstaq, B. et al. Reduced glutathione and S-acetylglutathione as selective apoptosis-inducing agents in cancer therapy. Found in: http://www.ncbi.nlm.nih.gov/pubmed/9018082

[5] Cuadrado, Ana, et al. Aplidin™ Induces Apoptosis in Human Cancer Cells via Glutathione Depletion and Sustained Activation of the Epidermal Growth Factor Receptor, Src, JNK, and p38 MAPK Found In: http://www.jbc.org/content/278/1/241.long

Chapter 19

[1] Hyman, Mark. Glutathione: The Mother of All Antioxidants. Found in:
http://www.huffingtonpost.com/dr-mark-hyman/glutathione-the-mother-of_b_530494.html

2 Performance nutrients. Found in:
http://www.livonlabs.com/cgi-bin/start.cgi/liposome-encapsulated/lypo-spheric-gsh.html

REFERENCES

Internet

Avitabile, M, et al. Correlation between serum glutathione reductases and bone densitometry values. Found in:
http://www.ncbi.nlm.nih.gov/pubmed/1821134

Balendiran, GK. The role of glutathione in cancer. Found In:
http://www.ncbi.nlm.nih.gov/pubmed/15386533

Barbagall, Mario, et al. Effects of Glutathione on Red Blood Cells Intracellular Magnesium. Found In:
http://hyper.ahajournals.org/content/34/1/76.full

Blankenber, Stefan, et al. Glutathione Peroxidase 1 Activity and Cardiovascular Events in Patients with Coronary Artery Disease Found in:
http://www.nejm.org/doi/full/10.1056/NEJMoa030535

Bounous, Gustavo, John Molson. The Antioxidant System. Found In:
http://www.getimmunocal.com/IMMTOP/Diseases/Cancer/The%20Antioxidant%20System.pdf

Bounous, Gustavo, John Molson. The Antioxidant System. Found In:
http://www.getimmunocal.com/IMMTOP/Diseases/Cancer/The%20Antioxidant%20System.pdf

Bowden, Johnny. "The Great Cholesterol Myth" Found in: http://www.youtube.com/watch?v=YGOpjPNtjes

Brown L., et al. "Chronic ethanol ingestion and the risk of acute lung injury: a role for glutathione availability?. Found In:

http://www.alcoholjournal.org/article/S0741-8329(04)00104-1/abstract

Buckley, BJ, et al. Regulation of endothelial cell prostaglandin synthesis by glutathione. Found In: http://www.ncbi.nlm.nih.gov/pubmed/1885596

Chatterjee, Anupam. Reduced Glutathione: A Radioprotector or a Modulator of DNA-Repair Activity? Found in: http://www.google.com.mx/url?sa=tandrct=jandq=andesrc=sandfrm=1andsource=webandcd=5andved=0CFYQFjAEandurl=http%3A%2F%2Fwww.mdpi.com%2F2072-6643%2F5%2F2%2F525%2Fpdfandei=VIuHUq_zNoTHiwLlg4HICgandusg=AFQjCNGGoiHI7NCTbnUiIEtJk73_F0Jo8g

Cuadrado, Ana, et al. Aplidin™ Induces Apoptosis in Human Cancer Cells via Glutathione Depletion and Sustained Activation of the Epidermal Growth Factor Receptor, Src, JNK, and p38 MAPK Found In: http://www.jbc.org/content/278/1/241.long

Cuadrado, Ana, et al. Aplidin™ Induces Apoptosis in Human Cancer Cells via Glutathione Depletion and Sustained Activation of the Epidermal Growth Factor Receptor, Src, JNK, and p38 MAPK Found In: http://www.jbc.org/content/278/1/241.long

Donnerstaq, B. et al. Reduced glutathione and S-acetylglutathione as selective apoptosis-inducing agents in cancer therapy. Found in: http://www.ncbi.nlm.nih.gov/pubmed/9018082

Dringen, R. Metabolism and functions of glutathione in brain. Found in:
http://www.ncbi.nlm.nih.gov/pubmed/10880854

Dringen, Ralf. Metabolism and functions of glutathione in brain. Found in:
http://members.shaw.ca/duncancrow/GSH-metabolism-in-brain.pdf

Dumaswala, UJ, et al. Glutathione protects chemo-kine scavenging and antioxidative defense functions in RBCs. Found in:
http://www.ncbi.nlm.nih.gov/pubmed/11245604

Ejaz ul Islam, Xiao-e Yang, [...], and Qaisar Mahmood. Assessing potential dietary toxicity of heavy metals in selected vegetables and food crops. Found in:
http://www.ncbi.nlm.nih.gov/pmc/articles/PMC1764924/

Fidelus, Rk, et al. Modulation of intracellular glutathione concentrations alters lymphocyte activation and proliferation. Found In:
http://www.ncbi.nlm.nih.gov/pubmed/3595735

Florian, S., et al. Cellular and subcellular localization of gastrointestinal glutathione peroxidase in normal and malignant human intestinal tissue. Found in:

http://www.ncbi.nlm.nih.gov/pubmed/11811519

Garcion, E, New clues about vitamin D functions in the nervous system. Found In:
http://www.ncbi.nlm.nih.gov/pubmed/11893522

Goto, I. Relation between reduced glutathione content and Heinz body formation in sheep erythrocytes. Found In: http://www.ncbi.nlm.nih.gov/pubmed/8484585

Guildford, Tim, MD. What Every Doctor Should Know About Glutathione. Found In: http://holisticprimarycare.net/topics/topics-o-z/vitamins-a-supplements/1421-what-every-doctor-should-know-about-glutathione.html

Hyman, Mark. Glutathione: The Mother of All Antioxidants. Found in: http://www.huffingtonpost.com/dr-mark-hyman/glutathione-the-mother-of_b_530494.html

Kidd, P. Th1/Th2 balance: the hypothesis, its limitations, and implications for health and disease. Found In: http://www.ncbi.nlm.nih.gov/pubmed/12946237

Lean, JM, et al. 'Normal skeletal development and regulation of bone formation and resorption'. Found in: http://www.uptodate.com/contents/normal-skeletal-development-and-regulation-of-bone-formation-and-resorption/abstract/100

Lean, JM, et al. 'Normal skeletal development and regulation of bone formation and resorption' Found in: http://www.uptodate.com/contents/normal-skeletal-development-and-regulation-of-bone-formation-and-resorption/abstract/96

Loquercui, C. The role of glutathione in the gastrointestinal tract: a review. Found in: http://www.ncbi.nlm.nih.gov/pubmed/10470601

http://www.medindia.net/facts/index.asp?pages 1- 10

Lundell, Dwight. Dr. Dwight Lundell on taking statins.
Found in: http://www.realfarmacy.com/world-renown-heart-surgeon-speaks-out-on-what-really-causes-heart-disease/

Mercola, Joseph. The Cholesterol Myth That Is Harming
Your Health. Found In:
http://articles.mercola.com/sites/articles/archive/2010/08/10/making-sense-of-your-cholesterol-numbers.aspx

Rouzer, C.A., et al. Depletion of glutathione selectively
inhibits synthesis of leukotriene C by macrophages.
Found in:
http://www.ncbi.nlm.nih.gov/pmc/articles/PMC31938 2/

Santangelo,F, et al. Restoring glutathione as a
therapeutic strategy in chronic kidney disease. Found in:
http://www.diagnose-me.com/cond/C15891.html

Santangelo, Francesco, et al. Restoring glutathione as a
therapeutic strategy in chronic kidney disease. Found in:
http://ndt.oxfordjournals.org/content/19/8/1951.full

Schnelldorfer, T. et al. Glutathione depletion causes cell
growth inhibition and enhanced apoptosis in pancreatic
cancer cells. Found in:
http://www.ncbi.nlm.nih.gov/pubmed/11013356

Sears, Barry. Another new wrinkle in the cholesterol
story. Found in:
http://zonediet.com/blog/2011/06/another-new-wrinkle-in-the-cholesterol-story/

Sidler, D., et al. Thiazolide-induced apoptosis in
colorectal cancer cells is mediated via the Jun kinase–Bim

axis and reveals glutathione-S-transferase P1 as Achilles' heel. Found in:
http://www.nature.com/onc/journal/v31/n37/abs/onc2011575a.html

Steinert, JR., et al. Nitric oxide signaling in brain function, dysfunction, and dementia. Found in:
http://www.ncbi.nlm.nih.gov/pubmed/20817920

About Enzymes. Found in:
http://www.anathenature.com/index.php?lay=showandac=articleandId=456355

BBC: Malhotra, A. Saturated fat heart disease "myth".
http://www.bbc.co.uk/news/health-24625808

Lifesaving Glutathione. Found In:
http://hwifc.com/glutathione/

[2] US Vitamin Injections Explains Glutathione Benefits in Brand New Article. Found In:
http://www.prnewswire.com/news-releases/us-vitamin-injections-explains-glutathione-benefits-in-brand-new-article-187449691.html

Performance nutrients. Found in:
http://www.livonlabs.com/cgi-bin/start.cgi/liposome-encapsulated/lypo-spheric-gsh.html

Prostaglandin. Found in:
http://en.wikipedia.org/wiki/Prostaglandin

What is the Role of Th1 and Th2 in Autoimmune Disease? Found In:
http://autoimmunepaleo.wordpress.com/2013/01/21/what-is-the-role-of-th1-and-th2-in-autoimmune-disease/

YOUTUBE: Harvard Profession Reveals the Truth about the Cholesterol Myth. Found in:
http://www.youtube.com/watch?v=iyB5Ylaf_w8

Made in the USA
Las Vegas, NV
20 April 2023